Coping Power

✓**Programs** *That Work*™

Coping Power

Parent Group Program

Workbook

Karen C. Wells • John E. Lochman • Lisa A. Lenhart

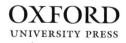

OXFORD

UNIVERSITY PRESS

2008

OXFORD
UNIVERSITY PRESS

Oxford University Press, Inc., publishes works that further
Oxford University's objective of excellence
in research, scholarship, and education.

Oxford   New York
Auckland   Cape Town   Dar es Salaam   Hong Kong   Karachi
Kuala Lumpur   Madrid   Melbourne   Mexico City   Nairobi
New Delhi   Shanghai   Taipei   Toronto

With offices in
Argentina   Austria   Brazil   Chile   Czech Republic   France   Greece
Guatemala   Hungary   Italy   Japan   Poland   Portugal   Singapore
South Korea   Switzerland   Thailand   Turkey   Ukraine   Vietnam

Copyright © 2008 by Oxford University Press, Inc.

Published by Oxford University Press, Inc.
198 Madison Avenue, New York, New York 10016

www.oup.com

Oxford is a registered trademark of Oxford University Press

ISBN 978-0-19-532796-0

About Programs *ThatWork*™

One of the most difficult problems confronting the parents of children with various disorders and diseases is finding the best help available. Everyone is aware of friends or family who have sought treatment from a seemingly reputable practitioner, only to find out later from another doctor that the original diagnosis was wrong or the treatments recommended were inappropriate or perhaps even harmful. Most parents or family members address this problem by reading everything they can about the children's symptoms, seeking out information on the Internet, or aggressively "asking around" to tap knowledge from friends and acquaintances. Governments and healthcare policymakers are also aware that people in need don't always get the best treatments—something they refer to as "variability in healthcare practices."

Now healthcare systems around the world are attempting to correct this variability by introducing "evidence-based practice." This simply means that it is in everyone's interest that patients of all ages get the most up-to-date and effective care for a particular problem. Healthcare policymakers have also recognized that it is very useful to give consumers of healthcare as much information as possible, so that they can make intelligent decisions in a collaborative effort to improve health and mental health. This series, Programs *ThatWork*™, is designed to accomplish just that for children suffering from behavioral health problems. Only the latest and most effective interventions for particular problems are described in user-friendly language. To be included in this series, each treatment program must pass the highest standards of evidence available, as determined by a scientific advisory board. Thus, when parents with children suffering from these problems or their family members seek out an expert clinician who is familiar with these interventions and decide that they are appropriate, they will have confidence that they are receiving the best care available. Of course, only your health care professional can decide on the right mix of treatments for your child.

This workbook is designed for you as a participant in the Coping Power Program. Over the course of two school years and 16 weekly group meetings, you will learn skills for effectively managing your child's aggressive behavior. You will learn techniques for eliminating misbehavior and positively reinforcing good behavior, as well as strategies for decreasing your stress through relaxation and time management.

All the materials necessary for successful completion of the Coping Power Program are provided in this workbook. It allows you to review the content of group meetings at home and reinforce what you learned in session so you can continue to use the skills you learn for many years to come.

David H. Barlow, Editor-in-Chief
Programs *ThatWork*™
Boston, Massachusetts

Contents

Coping Power Program—Schedule of Group Meetings

Session #	Date	Time	Location
1			
2			
3			
4			
5			
6			
7			
8			
9			
10			
11			
12			
13			
14			
15			
16			

Coping Power Parent Program
Year 1

Chapter 1

Session 1: Welcome!

Goals

- To learn about the Coping Power Program

- To meet the other members of your group

- To learn how you can provide your child with academic support in the home

The Coping Power Program

Welcome to the Coping Power Program! By participating in this program you are taking a positive and proactive approach to parenting. Over the course of the next two school years, you will work with qualified professionals to develop and refine skills that you can use to help your child cope with the transition to middle school.

Children naturally change as they grow up, and some of these changes can be difficult to cope with, both for children and their parents. One of the big changes that your child will face is the transition from elementary school to middle school. This transition often represents a real challenge for children and may be a stressful time for parents as well. Children must adjust to a new school setting and to having different teachers for each class, and they will have to learn to organize multiple homework assignments. They must change classes throughout the day, deal with increased expectations for self-responsibility and independence, and handle increasing peer pressure. Because of all of these adjustments and stresses, this time represents a major challenge to children's (and parents') coping abilities. Sometimes children may not know how to cope effectively with all of these stressors, and it would not be unusual to see an increase in academic and behavioral difficulties during this time period. Though it may come as a surprise to you, even children who have made it through their elementary school years with very few problems will likely experience difficulties.

The Coping Power Program is designed to teach children positive coping skills to prevent future difficulties that may otherwise occur. The program is also designed to assist you with developing and refining skills that can help support the coping skills that your child is learning in the group. In addition, the program emphasizes the use of parenting skills that may help to ward off behavioral difficulties that children may already be displaying or may display in the future. Even if your child is not currently having behavior problems, the skills taught in this program emphasize prevention and encourage healthy child development.

About the Child Group

Your child may have started to meet with a group at school. If so, he or she will be attending a total of 36 sessions on a weekly basis over the course of the fifth- and sixth-grade school years. Likewise, you will attend 16 parent group meetings during the same time period. Your group leader will provide you with a schedule of meetings. You may record the dates and times on the schedule found at the front of this workbook.

In the child group meetings, children will work on developing and improving their coping skills. The goal is to help the children learn skills that will help them make better choices, get along better with others, and manage negative emotions in an appropriate manner. Children are encouraged to set goals for themselves, and their group leader will track their progress in meeting them. If your child is participating in the Coping Power Program, he or she will be required to set weekly goals. Your child's teacher will monitor his or her progress in achieving goals by completing a Goal Sheet for your child every week. It will be your child's responsibility to bring this Goal Sheet to the teacher for sign-off. This sheet provides you with information as to whether or not your child has met the weekly goal.

About the Parent Group

As mentioned, parent group meetings will be held during your child's fifth- and sixth-grade years. There are a total of 16 sessions, in which you will be presented with various parenting skills and techniques. Sessions or meetings will consist of group discussion, along with exercises and role-play to illustrate certain techniques, particularly those related to communicating with your child and reinforcing positive behavior. In order to fully comprehend the concepts presented in group, it is important that you attend all sessions. Attendance is key to getting the most benefit from this group. Also important is completing your homework assignments. At the end of most sessions, your group leader will ask you to go home and practice what you have learned in that week's meeting. This workbook includes all the worksheets and forms you need to complete your homework.

Group Rules

The Number 1 rule of the group is confidentiality. It is an important part of the group process. Confidentiality means that your group leader will not share any information about you or the other parents to anyone outside the group. It also means that you should not talk about the other group members to anyone outside the group. In order to maintain group privacy and ensure that everyone feels comfortable discussing their problems or other issues during group meetings, we ask you to sign the following confidentiality statement.

As part of my group participation, I agree not to discuss outside of the group, anything regarding any parent or any child that is discussed in the group.

Signature: _____ Date: _____

Printed Name: _____

Additional rules include coming to all meetings on time and calling your group leader before the meeting if you are going to be late or absent. We recommend that you not miss any meetings, as each group session builds on material from the previous session. During group meetings there will often be group discussion. Please be considerate of other parents and refrain from interrupting when other members are speaking. Also, fighting, arguing, or other aggressive behavior will not be tolerated.

Getting to Know the Other Parents

In your first group session, you will be asked to pair up with another parent and conduct an interview. During this activity, try to find out enough information about the other parent to be able to introduce that person to the rest of the group. Ask about your partner's family, hobbies and interests, favorite foods and music, etc. Record your partner's responses in the space provided here.

_____

_____

_____

_____

_____

_____

_____

_____

Academic Support in the Home

The topic of this week's session is ways in which parents can provide academic support to their children, particularly when it comes to keeping up to date on children's homework assignments.

In order for parents to support their children's completion of homework, they have to be aware of what is happening at school. Parents need to have a method for keeping up to date on homework assignments and be able to monitor their child's progress effectively. Sometimes children mislead parents by telling them that they do not have homework or that they did it in school, when they actually did not. If there is an effective homework-monitoring system in place, some academic problems can be avoided. If not, it may be beneficial for you to set up a system with your child's teacher and enlist his help in establishing a method for monitoring homework. Simple techniques such as having a folder that includes the day's homework with a note written by the teacher at the end of each day may be all that is required. In this notebook would be a page on which your child writes down the assignment for every subject. At the end of the class period or the end of the day the teacher initials each assignment to indicate that it is listed correctly. The teacher should be asked to add anything that the child has left out and to let you know if your child has completed any of the homework during class time. In addition, the folder should have a parent signature page on which you would write comments or concerns and indicate whether or not your child completed the assignments.

You will learn more about creating a homework system during the next session. In the meantime, you may want to think about setting up a meeting with your child's teacher to discuss setting up a homework system, among other things. Following are some sample questions that you may want to ask your child's teacher.

- What is the daily classroom schedule for the children in your class?

- What are your classroom rules and expectations?

- What is your homework policy?

- Do children ever do homework in school or do you expect them to do all of it at home?

- If I get my child a homework assignment book, would you be willing to check it and initial it at the end of every day to make sure he has written down all assignments?

- Does the school have an automated or Web-based system that parents can use for accessing their child's homework assignments?

- How can I support my child in completing his or her homework at home?

- How is my child doing in school so far? How is he doing academically? How is his behavior?

- How often will you and I be communicating about my child? How often do you communicate with parents in general? How often would you be willing to communicate?

- What is your policy about receiving phone calls from parents?

- What can I do to be an involved parent?

- Other: _____

- Other: _____

- Other: _____

If you currently have concerns about your child's behavior or academic performance, try to set up a teacher meeting before the next group session.

Chapter 2

Session 2: Academic Support in the Home

Goals

- To set up a homework system and monitor your child's progress in completing school assignments

How to Set up a Good Homework System at Home

As discussed last week, there are a variety of things you can do to increase the likelihood that your child will complete his or her homework. One way to accomplish this is to establish a homework system that allows you to track your child's progress in completing assignments.

Homework is an opportunity for children to learn and for parents to be involved in their child's education. It is also an opportunity for parents to teach their child that learning can be fun and that education is important. When children know their parents care about homework, they have a good reason to complete and turn in their assignments.

Why Do Teachers Assign Homework?

Teachers assign homework for various reasons:

- To review and practice what has been taught in school
- To prepare for the next day's class
- To teach children how to use resources (library, reference books, etc.)
- To explore subjects in greater depth than time permits in class
- To teach children to work more independently
- To encourage self-discipline and responsibility

How Can You Help Your Child with Homework?

1. **Set expectations.** You must communicate clearly to your child what the expectations are for homework behavior. You may seek your child's input (your child may help determine the homework time or spot), and you should provide an opportunity for your child to ask questions. However, you must remain in charge of the homework process, even as the child remains responsible for the homework itself. As children become more responsible toward their homework, they may require less parental monitoring.

2. **Assist your child in bringing home assignments and necessary materials.**

   - Provide an adequate backpack or other method of carrying materials.

   - Provide the necessary assignment book.

   - Check what was brought home as early as possible.

3. **Identify a time and place where homework will be done each day.** Setting a consistent time for homework is a good idea. This time can be modified if necessary, but consistency is important. If your child is not used to completing homework during chunks of time, you may need to begin with setting 15 minutes as a goal and gradually increasing the time allotted to 45 minutes or an hour. As with time, it is a good idea to assign an area in which homework will be completed. This area should be organized so that homework can be accomplished there. This requires privacy, a writing surface, a place to store materials, and a place to put finished work so it will not be forgotten the next day (perhaps a backpack). The homework place does not have to be fancy, but should be in a quiet area and should remain consistent from day to day. A special box for materials along with an expectation that homework be done at the kitchen table is often all that is needed.

4. **Remove distractions.** Turn off the TV and radio, and do not allow social telephone calls. It helps if all family members can engage in quiet activities during homework time so that there

is not a lot of noisy distraction. If there are young children in the home who may be noisy, remove them from the homework area. If distractions cannot be eliminated, consider changing the location of the homework area (e.g., community library).

5. **Set a homework time.** Issues to be considered here include the following:

   ■ The child's schedule (e.g., most alert, fewest conflicting interests)

   ■ The family's schedule (e.g., parent's work schedule, dinner time)

   ■ Parent's personal schedule (e.g., meetings, activities, sleep)

   ■ Siblings' schedule (e.g., when are they most likely to not disrupt the child's homework time)

   ■ Potential distractions (e.g., favorite TV show, opportunity to play outside while still light, community activities that they would like to be involved in)

   ■ The amount of time required to complete homework

Note: *Some children actually focus better with some background noise, so you may need to individually tailor rules and structure.*

6. **Review assignments.** Check your child's assignment book or homework tracking form from school if there is one, and review your child's homework for the day. Or, check the school's homework Web page if there is one to see your child's assignments. At the beginning of each homework session, help your child set up each academic task, if this help is needed, and review the instructions with your child.

7. **Provide supplies.** Pencils, erasers, paper, dictionary, glue, stapler, calculator, pencil sharpener, scissors, and a ruler should all be kept nearby. Keep all supplies together in one place if possible. If you cannot provide supplies, check with the teacher, school counselor, or principal about sources of assistance.

8. **Set a total duration for homework** (e.g., 45 minutes). This rule should be standard unless there is a change in the normal rou-

tine. Modify the time in accordance with times when a lot of homework was assigned or only a small amount of homework is assigned. If your child works very hard but does not complete the assignments you must evaluate what is not working (e.g., is the teacher assigning too much homework? Is your child not working productively? Does your child have a specific problem that needs to be addressed [e.g., attention, reading])? Each problem will call for a different plan of action.

9. **Set a good example.** Read, write, or do other activities that require thought and effort.

10. **Show an interest.** Talk with your child about homework assignments. Take your child to the library for materials. Most importantly, read with your child.

11. **Vary the structure.** Whatever your child's age, if your child is having difficulty completing and turning in assignments that previously caused no difficulty, it is probably time to increase supervision and structure.

12. **Be available to help during homework time.** Being present during homework time has the advantage of increased monitoring and provides your child with a source of assistance and support. If you cannot be present during homework time, use resources available to you in your community to help (e.g., enroll your child in an after-school program, ask friends or neighbors to help, call home to check on your child's status, provide your child with small rewards for homework done in your absence).

Monitoring Homework

Children will differ with regard to the amount and intensity of monitoring they need to progress through their homework. For example, children who have learning disabilities or difficulty sustaining attention need more monitoring than other children. It is up to you to determine the best level of monitoring for your child.

As your child works, you should monitor her progress on a regular basis and make sure that you give praise for appropriate work behavior. Initially, for children this age, it may be necessary to monitor and offer praise every 15 minutes. As your child gets used to the new structure you can extend this period of time. You can offer help during these check-in times but assistance should be kept to a minimum so that your child remains focused on completing her work independently. If your child requires your help, offer it only after she has attempted all assignments.

An alternative to monitoring at specified time intervals is to help your child break daily homework assignments down into manageable pieces. For example, you can instruct your child to do her math homework first and then bring it to you for review. After you have reviewed the math assignment, your child can move on to the next piece of homework. After your child completes each homework assignment, she can bring it to you to be checked. Remember to offer praise for correct items and identify incorrect items. Do not scold or criticize your child for incorrect responses; simply tell your child which items are incorrect, and suggest that she go back and try to correct the wrong answers.

As mentioned, you may wish to also set a time limit for the completion of all homework (e.g., 45 minutes or an hour). Your child must be working the entire time before homework time can be over. If your child is unable to finish all assignments in the time allotted, you should consider whether the teacher assigned too much work or if your child was not working productively. Alternatively, if your child finishes before the allotted time, suggest that she read a book until the allotted time is over. This will discourage the tendency to rush through homework too quickly.

Working with Your Child

Regardless of how you choose to design your homework system, you should work closely with your child in developing it. Ask for your child's input on how the homework system should be designed so that it is easy for everybody involved (child, teacher, and parent). By allowing your child to give input into developing the program you provide a sense of "ownership" of the plan so that your child will be more motivated to follow it. Some areas in which children could be asked to give their input include the following:

- Exact time for homework

- Exact place for homework

- How frequently they would like parents to check their homework

- Color of notebook

- Whether or not the teacher should initial each entry or if they would like to do it on their own and see how it goes

Homework System Forms

At the end of the chapter are examples of forms that you may find helpful when setting up your homework system. Please feel free to photocopy them from the book or create forms of your own.

Homework

- Establish a homework system with your child and be ready to discuss it with the group at the next meeting.

- If you haven't done so already, you may want to set up a meeting with your child's teacher to discuss the homework system.

My Homework Plan

I, _____ , agree to the homework plan outlined below.

I will:

- Decide when and where I will do my homework. For example, I will pick a quiet place in the house and pick a time of day to always do my homework.

- Make sure I have all the things I need before starting my homework. For example, I will make sure that I have pencils, paper, erasers, or anything else I may need.

- Always put away everything else that I do not need

- Not do my homework in front of the television or while listening to the radio

- Not talk on the phone during the time I have put aside to complete my homework

- Work on big projects by breaking them down into smaller, more manageable pieces. I will work on the smaller pieces each day.

- Always double-check my answers

- Always ask mom or dad to check my homework and make sure that I have completed everything

- Place notes to remind myself of what I need to do. I will put these notes in a place where I will see them (e.g., my locker, notebook, or desk).

I will do my homework at _____ (time) and I will do it in the _____ (place). If I need to change this schedule, I will talk to mom or dad first.

I will ask _____ to check my homework when I am finished.

Signed: _____ Date: _____

Homework Tracking Form—Teacher Version

Dear parent,

Your child, _____, is missing the following assignments in:

Math (Teacher signature : _____)

_____

_____

Social Studies (Teacher signature : _____)

_____

_____

Language (Teacher signature : _____)

_____

_____

Science (Teacher signature : _____)

_____

_____

Health (Teacher signature : _____)

_____

_____

Reading (Teacher signature : _____)

_____

_____

Other _____ (Teacher signature : _____)

_____

_____

_____

Chapter 3

Session 3: Managing Your Stress—Part I

Goals

- To talk about stress and the impact it has on your life

- To learn the importance of time management and taking care of your personal needs

- To learn active relaxation

The Causes of Stress

Many people think of stress as being caused only by negative events or crises. Obvious examples include the death of a family member or someone close to you, physical injury, illness, and natural disasters. However, stress can also be caused by events that most people would think of as positive. For example, getting married, buying a home, relocating, or starting a new job are often highly stressful. Regardless of the cause, stress can sometimes build up to extreme levels.

What Is Stress?

Stress has to do with the physical reactions that take place in your body. When you are faced with difficult events to which you must adjust, your body may respond with a number of changes. Your heart rate and breathing rate may increase, your blood pressure may rise, your muscles may become tense and tight, your hands may feel cold and sweaty, or all of these things may happen at once. If you are already in a state of chronic stress, and then another stressor is added (e.g., your car breaks down, your child yells at you or is being very uncooperative), the chemicals in your brain may overreact, causing you to experience an emotional reaction that may be extreme. When your body is reacting and overreacting in this way you feel anxious, tired, and tense, and over a long period of time you can feel chronically fatigued or even physically sick.

Stress in Parenting

Parenting can be very stressful at times, especially if parents also have a number of other ongoing daily stressors in their lives. Children can be quite demanding of their parents' attention, and if they are having behavior or learning problems at home or at school, they may require extra energy, effort, and problem solving on the part of the parent. Such children present their parents with many situations that require some type of disciplinary action, creative solutions, or thoughtful, positive consequences. Parents may find that they must take themselves off "automatic pilot" in their reactions to their children and must constantly think through how they want to manage their child. While this kind of proactive approach is in the child's best interest, it can also be stressful for the parent, who must constantly be on the front line thinking, planning, and acting. When parents are also experiencing other stressful events in their lives, the possibility for emotional overreaction and loss of control in parent–child encounters increases.

Time Management

Most parents devote little time to themselves. Use the form on page 19 to help you visualize how you are prioritizing your time. It is not uncommon for people to be unaware of the demands on their time and the areas of their lives that they are neglecting.

Taking Care of Your Personal Needs

Think about some of the ways in which you can take care of your personal needs. What are some things you can do to better take care of yourself? Some examples include the following:

■ Reading a book

■ Listening to music

Pie Chart of Life

Use this page to create a pie chart in which each slice of the pie represents a part of your life. Write down all of the various roles you play, count them up, and divide the pie into that many slices. Make sure each slice is correctly sized to correspond to how much time and energy the role currently takes up in your life.

My Roles:

_____   _____   _____   _____

_____   _____   _____   _____

_____   _____   _____   _____

Ideally, there should be one piece of the pie that is devoted to taking care of yourself. However, for many parents, this piece of the pie gets smaller and smaller with the passage of time and the imposition of new responsibilities. The end result is often the complete neglect of self. You may think that you have to do this in order to meet the demands of the other roles in your life, but if you neglect yourself for too long, you will end up having little stamina, energy, or enthusiasm to give to those other areas of your life. Taking care of yourself is one of the first steps in stress management. It will help you feel better and be more effective in all areas of your life.

- Taking a warm bath

- Going for a leisurely walk

- Practicing meditation or yoga

For some parents, taking care of their personal needs may mean claiming 30 minutes out of the day for themselves when they first get home from work. Think about whether or not this will work for you. Keep in mind that these 30 minutes are meant for relaxation only. It is important that you put boundaries around this time and protect it from intrusion from other family members or other chores that need attention.

Use the worksheet provided to list activities you can do that can reduce stress and help you relax and how often you will try to do them. Also write down the arrangements that need to be made for you to be able to engage in these activities (e.g., hiring a babysitter, having your spouse cook dinner, etc.)

Active Relaxation

In addition to engaging in pleasurable activities, you can reduce stress through a technique called "active relaxation." Remember, stress affects the body in multiple ways (faster heart rate, high blood pressure, muscle tension) and often results in fatigue that negatively affects a person's ability to function. The effects of stress can also have a negative impact on your ability to parent because you may become too tired and have less energy to devote to parenting. If you can learn to manage stress during the day, you will be more able to find the time, energy, and interest needed to carry out the role of being an effective parent.

Use the following script to carry out active relaxation whenever you are feeling stressed.

Active Relaxation Script

Most people are not aware that when they are upset or agitated, one or more of their muscle groups are tense and their breathing is rapid

Taking Care of Myself Worksheet — homework

Activities that I will do to take care of myself   Frequency

- Long walks
- yoga
- warm bath
- listening to music

Arrangements that will need to be made during these times:

and shallow. If we can learn to control our muscle tension and our breathing, we can teach our bodies to stay relatively calm and relaxed, even in upsetting situations. The following is a procedure for achieving relaxation quickly. By practicing every day, within 2 to 3 weeks you will be able to relax your body by simply saying the word *relax* to yourself in real-life situations with your child and in other stressful situations.

1. *Get comfortable in your chair. Place your arms on the arms of the chair. Close your eyes and keep them closed throughout the entire exercise.*

2. *Become aware of the various muscle groups in your body (e.g., hands and arms; face, neck, and shoulders; chest and stomach; hips, legs, and feet).*

3. *Bend your arms at the elbow. Then, make a tight fist with both hands while tightening the biceps and forearms. Hold for 5 seconds. Pay attention to the tension. Then relax. Pay attention to the relaxation.*

4. *Tense your entire face and shoulders, tightly shut your eyes and wrinkle your forehead, pull the corners of mouth toward your ears, tighten your neck and hunch your shoulders. Hold for 5 seconds. Pay attention to the tension. Relax. Pay attention to the relaxation.*

5. *Take in a deep breath and arch your back. Hold this position for 5 seconds. Now relax. Take in another deep breath and press out your stomach. Hold . . . . and relax.*

6. *Raise your feet off the floor while keeping your knees straight. Pull your feet and toes back toward your face and tighten the muscles in your shins. Hold . . . and relax. Now, curl your toes down toward the floor, tighten your calves, thighs and buttocks and hold . . . . and relax.*

7. *Scan each muscle group in your mind and relax any tense muscles.*

8. *Now, become aware of your breathing. Slow your breathing down as you breathe in and out, in and out.*

9. *With your next deep breath, count slowly from 1 to 5 as you breathe in and count from 6 to 10 as you breathe out. Your stomach should expand and deflate with each breath.*

10. *Repeat this deep, slow, breathing . . . . in and out . . . . . in and out . . . . Stop when you are feeling deeply relaxed.*

11. *Say the word "relax" to yourself approximately 20 times every time you exhale.*

12. *Now, gradually let your breathing return to normal and open your eyes.*

Homework

✎ If not done during the session, complete the Taking Care of Myself Worksheet and begin engaging in the enjoyable activities listed.

✎ Practice active relaxation one to two times each day until the next session.

Chapter 4

Session 4: Managing Your Stress—Part II

Goals

■ To explore ways to manage stress in daily life

■ To learn about the cognitive model of stress and mood management

Managing Stressful Events and Daily Hassles

This week's topic involves steps you can take to manage stress in your life. One approach has to do with managing the multitude of daily hassles that are a part of every person's life. Although we cannot always control whether or not we experience stressful events, we can exert some control over how we manage them. For people who experience a lot of stress, it may be necessary for them to list the stressors and then prioritize them, starting with those that require immediate attention and ending with those that can be dealt with at a later date. One option is to list all the things that need to be done in a specific period of time (e.g., a week), then prioritize them by importance, and make a plan to meet your goals within that week. Remember, most things take twice as long as you think they will to complete. Leave enough time so that small "emergencies" can be taken care of without steering you off track.

Putting Time Where It Belongs

At times people experience stress because they do not pay attention to how they are handling or juggling different roles and expectations. The following guidelines provide useful ideas for managing stress more effectively.

Know What Needs to be Done and Learn to Prioritize

Know your goals and when they need to be met. A day planner, calendar, or other device that allows you to write out what you need to get done is usually helpful. Set timelines that allow for small "emergencies" (sometimes called "wiggle room"). This will help to reduce stress by giving you some leeway within your schedule.

Block Your Time

If you find yourself with many tasks that require small amounts of time or can be done simultaneously, do them together. For example, you may be able to do laundry, clean the oven (self-clean), and conduct a conference call all at the same time. Alternatively, if you need to run short errands, make sure that you do these in a planned manner (map out your course of action to reduce wasted time).

Set Realistic Goals

Do not overburden yourself. Know your limits and set goals that you know you can achieve. There is, however, a delicate balance between setting the bar too high (setting unrealistically high goals) and setting it too low (not setting enough goals). If you do not set your goals high enough, there is the chance that stress will increase. Not only will you fail to get your jobs done, but the lack of activity and lack of success in meeting goals will have a negative effect on your functioning. Know your limits, but take them to their end!

Juggle Tasks

Life comes with many surprises, both good and bad, and these surprises usually put our schedules off course, resulting in frantic attempts to catch up. This action of frantically trying to catch up is usually ineffective and typically results in feeling stressed out. So, instead of trying to catch up, accept the change and look at your list and identify low-priority items that can be moved to a different day or different week. This is why you prioritize in writing. You can easily identify what can be put off and you can make sure that it is rescheduled.

Improve Energy Level

Low energy can be the result of illness, poor eating habits, sleep deprivation, being overloaded with work or chores, and many other things. It is important to look for the source of the decreased energy and find a solution. Try eating right, getting enough sleep, and working hours that allow you to rest and enjoy part of every day. People often think that "burning the midnight oil" will help reduce stress because "at least one job is complete." However, this often backfires because the next thing on the list becomes a priority and the cycle of overwork, lack of sleep, and poor eating continues. A healthy lifestyle will lead to increased energy, and this energy in turn will help you to meet your goals.

Get Rid of Environmental Chaos!

There are few things as stressful as a disorganized, cluttered, and dirty life space. Unfortunately, with the demands of work, parenting, and other roles, it is difficult to keep our environments neat and clean. While the ultimate goal would be to keep "everything" clean, try setting goals to work on one room at a time and set a schedule for cleaning. Enlist the help of your spouse and children and make sure to reward yourself for the completion of goals. Though it is oftentimes impossible to do (financially), hiring someone to clean and organize your household can reduce stress substantially. Not only does this help provide hours that can be put toward other things (e.g., being with family, taking care of yourself), but you no longer have to carry out jobs that are generally considered unpleasant. Also, good organization makes it easier to do your jobs—you know where things are and do not have to waste time searching for things.

Schedule Time for Yourself Each Day

Make sure that each day you set aside "personal time." This may be on your lunch break, before work, or after work—the time should be set according to what fits in *your* schedule, not someone else's! Be sure to make the time substantial enough to give you a feeling of being rested, but not so long that it interferes with your ability to meet your other goals. Remember, the key to stress management is to be able to handle multiple tasks and keep in control of your time. If you put too much time into any one thing, other areas will suffer.

Schedule Time off Weekly, Monthly, and Yearly

Do not assume that other people will make sure that you keep time for personal use—you need to plan ahead. This time is in addition to the time you take each day. These segments should be longer and be used for doing enjoyed activities. Vacations can be as short or as long as you want, just plan ahead and make sure that you do not schedule important tasks just before you leave or just after you come back. Everyone needs time to readjust to the needs of home and work and you should plan for this.

Just Say No

Saying "no" or setting limits with people takes practice and planning. In part, your ability to say no will improve when you are clear about your priorities. If you have a high-priority event or task that you need to accomplish and someone asks you to do something for them, you already know that your time is allocated and you can't help out. This does not mean that you need to practice being rude. On the contrary, people appreciate it if you set your priorities and do not accept tasks that you cannot complete or will complete in a haphazard fashion while under duress. Know your limits and be assertive when people are trying to get you to overextend yourself.

Stop Procrastinating

The old adage "Don't put off to tomorrow what you can do today" is applicable here. Achieving your goals and giving yourself rewards for doing so is a great stress reducer!

Cognitive Model of Stress and Mood Management

Your thoughts are very important in managing your reactions to stress. They can contribute to how stressed or upset you feel, and they can also reduce the impact that stress has on your life. Usually, the sequence of thinking, feeling, and reacting goes like this:

- Something happens

- You have a thought or thoughts about the event

- These thoughts create a feeling, either positive or negative

- You act or behave in ways that reflect those feelings

For example, Ms. Watson went to the dentist's office and arrived promptly at her scheduled appointment time. Unfortunately, she was left waiting in the office for over 2 hours without any word from office personnel. Ms. Watson believed that the dentist had purposely left her waiting because he was angry with her for missing her previous appointment without calling to cancel. The first thought that ran through her mind was that her dentist was a mean and vengeful person and that he deserved to be punished for his behavior. After having this thought she became very angry, yelled at the receptionist, and stormed out of the office.

Think about this example and come up with a different scenario using positive thoughts. For example, if Ms. Watson had believed that her dentist was running late because he was involved in a difficult procedure that was scheduled on an emergency basis, she probably would not have thought of him as mean or vengeful. She might also have stayed at the office and had her procedure completed, or she might have chosen to reschedule her appointment.

According to the cognitive model of stress and mood management, people act very differently according to their thoughts about a situation. These thoughts are called "automatic thoughts," or ATs, which seem to happen instantly and without much reflection. In Ms. Watson's situation, she could have prevented her angry outburst by simply speaking with the receptionist and asking questions in a calm manner. Even if she did not like the information given to her, the fact that she asked a question and maintained emotional control would have helped her to get her needs met in the most effective manner. The saying "Ask, don't assume" is a good one to remember, because in many situations it is our assumptions that mislead us and result in interpersonal problems or increased stress.

When you find yourself experiencing negative thoughts and feelings about a particular situation, it can be helpful to put things in writing. Take a look at the sample Thoughts, Feelings, and Behavior Worksheet on page 31.

Try to remember a time when you experienced negative thoughts and feelings in a situation with your child that resulted in an extreme reaction on your part. Also think about a time when your positive thoughts about a situation with your child led to behavior that was justified by the situation. For example, say your child breaks a precious lamp while helping you vacuum the house. If your automatic thought at the time is, "It was only an accident, my child was only trying to help me," you would let go of your anger and assure your child that you are not upset and that you understand he or she didn't break the lamp on purpose.

Use the blank Thoughts, Feelings, and Behavior Worksheet on page 32 to list one or two personal examples of instances in which some event, and the thoughts associated with it, led to a negative reaction or overreaction on your part. We have also included a list of feeling words that you may choose from when filling out the worksheet. It is common for people to use the same word to describe very different feelings. For example, there are varying degrees of anger. You may be slightly annoyed or furious. It is important to make distinctions.

Homework

✎ If not completed during the session, fill out the Thoughts, Feelings, and Behavior Worksheet before the next meeting.

✎ Continue to use stress management techniques and modify your plan for taking care of yourself as necessary.

Thoughts, Feelings, and Behavior Worksheet

Dysfunctional Thought Sequence

Thoughts	Feelings	Behavior
My child is doing this on purpose to hurt me	Enraged	Screaming at or hitting my child
My child just does not care about me	Depressed	Give up trying to help my child
My child is just bad and there is nothing I can do to change that	Hopeless	Withdraw attention from my child
I must be a bad parent for my child to act like this	Guilty and inadequate	Reward my child for negative behavior

Functional Thought Sequence

Thoughts	Feelings	Behavior
My child's intentions are good but he can't always control his behavior	Loving and determined	Kind but firm response to disruptive behavior
My child loves me even though his behavior is sometimes bad	Happy and secure	Good follow-through with parenting skills that will help my child
My child's behavior can improve with my help	Determined and understanding	Pay attention to my child's positive behavior
I am a good parent	Competent	Act loving and firm

Figure 4.1

Example of Completed Thoughts, Feelings, and Behavior Worksheet

Thoughts, Feelings, and Behavior Worksheet

Dysfunctional Thought Sequence

Thoughts	Feelings	Behavior

Functional Thought Sequence

Thoughts	Feelings	Behavior

Feeling Words

Happiness	Pleased	Ashamed
Joy	Relaxed	Guilty
Irritated	Angered	Euphoric
Depressed	Anxious	Tense
Sadness	Fearful	Uptight
Incompetent	Scared	Calm
Frustrated	Dread	Aggravated
Grief	Apprehensive	Confused
Annoyed	Worried	Perturbed
Enraged	Tired	Solemn
Inadequate	Bored	Isolated
Cheerful	Gloomy	Overwhelmed
Excited	Worthless	Nervous

Chapter 5

Session 5: Basic Social Learning Theory and Improving the Parent–Child Relationship

Goals

- To learn about social learning theory and the ABC model

- To begin tracking and labeling your child's behavior

- To come up with activities that you and your child can do together

Social Learning Theory

If your child is participating in the Coping Power Program at school, she is currently learning skills that can be used to control her own behavior, cope with anger, and interact appropriately with peers and teachers. These skills are based on social learning theory, a theory that says that behavior is influenced by the events that occur just before and just after it. For example, children in this age range often pay very close attention to how their parents react when they do something. As such, your behavior has a lot to do with whether your child will display that behavior again in the future. Because of your role as a parent, you can do a lot to help your child improve positive behavior and decrease negative behavior.

ABC Model

From this point on in the program, the group will talk a lot about children's behavior. *Behavior* is represented by the letter *B* on the ABC model (see Fig. 5.1). A behavior is something observable that a child does. It can be good or bad. For example, walking, screaming, arguing, hitting, and washing the dishes are all behaviors.

The *A* on the model refers to *antecedents* and the *C* refers to *consequences*. Antecedents are the events that happen just before a child's

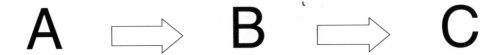

ANTECEDENTS   BEHAVIOR   CONSEQUENCES

Figure 5.1

ABC Model of Social Learning Theory

behavior, and consequences are the events that happen just after it. These events have a lot to do with how you can control your child's behavior.

Positive Consequences for Good Behavior

You can modify your child's behavior by using positive consequences to reward good behavior. Research has shown that if children receive positive consequences for their good behavior, they are more likely to repeat that behavior in the future. The consequence should occur as close to the behavior a possible; this increases the likelihood that the child will make the connection that their behavior resulted in this consequence. Examples of positive consequences include things like trips to the store, getting a movie, going out for ice cream, etc. Sometimes parents give these treats "free of charge"—that is, they don't require anything of the child first. However, to function as a positive consequence, it is necessary to communicate to the child that these special treats or activities are being given because the child displayed some specific good behavior(s). Without specifically making that connection, the special treat will not function to help improve the child's behavior. Of course, this also means that if the child does not perform the specified behavior(s), the parents must withhold the special treat until the child does perform the behavior(s). You may have to learn to manage tantrums or negative emotional reactions from your child the first few times you withhold treats from her.

In addition to special treats, activities, or outings, praise can also be used as a positive consequence or reinforcer. Praising your child increases the likelihood that your child will exhibit good behavior, and it will improve her self-esteem.

Praise

Praise should be given at the time your child exhibits a good behavior. It is okay to offer praise long after the behavior has occurred, but it is important to note that immediate praise is more effective than delayed praise. Try to remember the phrase, "catch my child being good." If you happen to forget to praise your child right away or if you notice something praiseworthy after the fact, it does not mean you should not praise your child. Praise can be given at any time, although it is always better to do it earlier rather than later.

There are two types of praise that parents can give.

- *Labeled praise* identifies exactly what your child did that was good. For example, "I like the way you completed your homework before dinner" is an example of labeled praise.

- *Unlabeled praise* indicates to the child that they did something well but does not say exactly what the behavior was. For example, "good job" is an example of unlabeled praise.

Both types of praise are effective and each may be more or less appropriate to any given situation. Labeled praise may be better if your child is having a hard time learning or displaying a new good behavior.

The Power of Praise

- Tell your child when you are proud of them.

- Use the words "thank you" as often as you would like to hear it back.

- Thank your child for behaving in positive or prosocial ways.

- Say, "You did a good job" *every time* you see your child doing something that is good.

- Tell your child that you appreciate them TRYING to follow the rules. If they do follow the rules, praise them again!

- Let your child know that you love them for who they are.

Tell them! Children are not mind readers; they need to hear praise directly from you.

Tracking Positive and Negative Behavior

In order to use positive consequences effectively, you need to be aware of your child's behavior. Often parents overlook good behavior, but are quick to notice bad behavior.

Take a look at the Child Behavior Checklist on page 39. The checklist is set up so that the positive behaviors in the right-hand column are opposite the negative behaviors in the left-hand column. Review the behaviors listed and check off those that are problematic for your child. If there are any negative behaviors that are a problem and are not on this list, add them in the space titled "Other." After you have checked all the negative behaviors, go back and select the three that are most problematic and identify them with the numbers 1, 2, and 3, accordingly.

Tracking and Praising Your Child's Behavior

Now that you have selected two or three negative behaviors and their good-behavior opposites, it is time to keep track of these behaviors using the Behavior Tracking Form, found at the end of the chapter. Every time your child does any of the negative or positive behaviors you've selected, circle the word *Observed* on the tracking form for the day that you saw it. If you praised the positive behavior, circle the word *Praised* on the form for the day that you provided praise. Do this for 2 weeks and bring your completed tracking forms to the next group meeting.

As discussed, there are two types of praise statements you can use:

Labeled Praise

Labeled praise is a praise statement that states exactly what the good behavior is. Examples are:

- "You did a good job of taking out the garbage when I asked you to."

- "Thank you for playing nicely with your little brother for 30 minutes."

Choose few negative behaviours ~~you~~ I might ignore.
Choose few positive behaviours I might enforce.
(Our pact)

Child Behavior Checklist

Negative Behavior

- [x] Argues
- [ ] Cries if doesn't his get way

- [x] Defies authority
- [ ] Destroys property
- [ ] Is fearful (inappropriately)
- [ ] Fights with siblings
- [ ] Fire setting
- [x] Hits others
- [ ] Hyperactive
- [ ] Irritable

- [ ] Lies
- [ ] Noisy
- [ ] Does not mind adults
- [ ] Does not eat meals
- [ ] Pouts
- [ ] Stays out too late
- [ ] Steals
- [ ] Talks back to adults
- [ ] Teases others
- [ ] Throws temper tantrums
- [ ] Whines
- [x] Yells
- [x] Gets in trouble at school
- [ ] Other ____
- [ ] Other ____

Positive Behavior

- [x] Discusses things calmly; accepts adult decisions
- [ ] Doesn't cry; discusses things calmly
- [x] Follows directions; obeys rules
- [ ] Uses objects appropriately
- [ ] Brave; assertive
- [ ] Plays and shares with siblings; assists them
- [ ] Does not play with fire
- [x] Solves problems verbally
- [x] Behaves calmly
- [ ] Concentrates
- [ ] Good natured; easy going
- [ ] Is honest
- [ ] Quiet; still; peaceful
- [x] Follows directions; accepts decisions
- [ ] Good appetite
- [x] Handles disappointments
- [ ] Obeys curfew
- [ ] Respects others' property
- [x] Is respectful; listens
- [x] Compliments others; doesn't insult others
- [x] Accepts "no"; negotiates well
- [ ] Uses age-appropriate voice
- [ ] Uses normal voice volume
- [x] Performs well in school
- [ ] Other ____
- [ ] Other ____

■ "I like the way you got your homework done on time tonight."

Unlabeled Praise

Unlabeled praise is a praise statement that tells the child their behavior was good, but it does not specify the exact behavior that was noticed. Examples are:

■ "Good job."

■ "Thank you."

■ "I like that."

Remember, both types of praise are good, but labeled praise is better if the child is having a hard time learning or displaying a new good behavior.

Parent–Child Special Time

In addition to praising good behaviors, it is also important that you spend relaxed, non-problem-focused time with your child. Even though your child is getting older, you are still the most important person in her life. You are the person your child looks to in times of stress, and you are the role model for her behavior. If you and your child have developed a positive relationship with one another and you nourish this relationship on a regular basis, it is more likely that your child will continue to look to you for support in the future. Maintaining a close, positive contact with your child is an excellent way to counteract the influence of negative outside forces. Such forces include but are not limited to peer groups (gang or other), the media, and negative adult role models. Research has shown that children who maintain close bonds to and positive relationships with their parents are less likely to join gangs, are less likely to be influenced by negative peer groups, and are more able to stand firm against negative peer pressure.

Maintaining a positive relationship with your child can often be accomplished with something as simple as making sure that you reserve 10 or 15 minutes per day to be with your child in a relaxed way, without a lot of other distractions. For example, you could spend 15 minutes a day talking with your child about her day. Ask about school, ask about plans for the week, and simply show an interest in what she is doing. You may want to spend those 15 minutes a day doing an activity together (e.g., playing a game) and talking with one another. In addition, some children this age still like to have their parents read to them, and this is a good way to nourish a close bond between parent and child. The main idea is that the time you spend with your child should not be used for discussing problems or negative behavior; this time should be protected and used only for positive interactions.

Think creatively about some activities that you and your child can do together. Think about things that your child would enjoy, not activities that need to be done for the family (e.g., chores, shopping for groceries, walking the family dog). Write down some of your ideas in the space provided.

_____

_____

_____

_____

_____

Keeping Special Time Special

It is important to note that this time is for *interaction* and not simply sharing the same physical space (e.g., watching TV together). It is important that children be interested and involved when spending time with parents. You need to encourage your child to talk and relate to you positively when you are sharing special time together. Ways to accomplish this include the following:

- Praise your child often

- Show an interest—ask questions

- Do not criticize or reprimand, regardless of what happens

- Defer all problems to a later time

- Avoid controversial subjects

- Have fun just being together

- Allow your child to choose the activity

- Participate fully in whatever activity your child chooses

Choosing an Activity

Pick an activity that you would like to engage in with your child. Set a goal for the number of times per week that you would like to spend interacting positively with your child. Be realistic about frequency and length of time allotted for this activity. For example, a good start would be to share special time with your child for 10 or 15 minutes a day three or four times per week.

Use the Special Time Worksheet provided to monitor your special time. The first line is for you to set a goal regarding frequency (e.g., three times per week for 1 hour; once a day for 20 minutes). For each day, list the activities and the time you spent interacting with your child. Keep track of any observations you may make during special time and record them in the space provided at the bottom of the worksheet.

Homework

✎ Complete the Behavior Tracking Form at the end of this chapter for 2 weeks (two copies are provided). Remember to praise your child's positive behavior.

✎ Begin spending special time with your child and complete the Special Time Worksheet.

Special Time Worksheet

My goal for this week is to: _____

DAY OF THE WEEK	SPECIAL TIME ACTIVITY (Please check all that apply and indicate type of activity you engaged in with your child)
SUNDAY	☐ At least 15 minutes talking ☐ Activity 1: _____ Time spent together: _____ ☐ Activity 2: _____ Time spent together: _____ ☐ Activity 3: _____ Time spent together: _____
MONDAY	☐ At least 15 minutes talking ☐ Activity 1: _____ Time spent together: _____ ☐ Activity 2: _____ Time spent together: _____ ☐ Activity 3: _____ Time spent together: _____
TUESDAY	☐ At least 15 minutes talking ☐ Activity 1: _____ Time spent together: _____ ☐ Activity 2: _____ Time spent together: _____ ☐ Activity 3: _____ Time spent together: _____
WEDNESDAY	☐ At least 15 minutes talking ☐ Activity 1: _____ Time spent together: _____ ☐ Activity 2: _____ Time spent together: _____ ☐ Activity 3: _____ Time spent together: _____
THURSDAY	☐ At least 15 minutes talking ☐ Activity 1: _____ Time spent together: _____ ☐ Activity 2: _____ Time spent together: _____ ☐ Activity 3: _____ Time spent together: _____

continued

Special Time Worksheet *continued*

DAY OF THE WEEK	SPECIAL TIME ACTIVITY (Please check all that apply and indicate type of activity you engaged in with your child)
FRIDAY	☐ At least 15 minutes talking ☐ Activity 1: _____ Time spent together: _____ ☐ Activity 2: _____ Time spent together: _____ ☐ Activity 3: _____ Time spent together: _____
SATURDAY	☐ At least 15 minutes talking ☐ Activity 1: _____ Time spent together: _____ ☐ Activity 2: _____ Time spent together: _____ ☐ Activity 3: _____ Time spent together: _____

Observations: _____

_____

_____

_____

_____

_____

_____

_____

_____

_____

_____

_____

Behavior Tracking Form

BEHAVIOR	Monday	Tuesday	Wednesday	Thursday	Friday	Saturday	Sunday
Neg: *Argues, talks back to adults*	Observed	Observed	Observed	Observed	Observed	Observed	Observed
Pos: *Discusses things calmly*	Observed Praised	Observed Praised	Observed Praised	Observed Praised	Observed Praised	Observed Praised	Observed Praised
Neg: *Defies authority*	Observed	Observed	Observed	Observed	Observed	Observed	Observed
Pos: *Follow directions, obeys rules*	Observed Praised	Observed Praised	Observed Praised	Observed Praised	Observed Praised	Observed Praised	Observed Praised
Neg: *Talks back to adults, Hits others*	Observed	Observed	Observed	Observed	Observed	Observed	Observed
Pos: *Solves problems verbally*	Observed Praised	Observed Praised	Observed Praised	Observed Praised	Observed Praised	Observed Praised	Observed Praised

Behavior Tracking Form

BEHAVIOR	Monday	Tuesday	Wednesday	Thursday	Friday	Saturday	Sunday
Neg: _____ _____	Observed	Observed	Observed	Observed	Observed	Observed	Observed
Pos: _____ _____	Observed Praised	Observed Praised	Observed Praised	Observed Praised	Observed Praised	Observed Praised	Observed Praised
Neg: _____ _____	Observed	Observed	Observed	Observed	Observed	Observed	Observed
Pos: _____ _____	Observed Praised	Observed Praised	Observed Praised	Observed Praised	Observed Praised	Observed Praised	Observed Praised
Neg: _____ _____	Observed	Observed	Observed	Observed	Observed	Observed	Observed
Pos: _____ _____	Observed Praised	Observed Praised	Observed Praised	Observed Praised	Observed Praised	Observed Praised	Observed Praised

Chapter 6

Session 6: Ignoring Minor Disruptive Behavior

Goals

- ▦ To learn how to ignore your child's minor disruptive behavior

- ▦ To continue tracking your child's behavior and begin monitoring your use of the ignoring technique

Ignoring Minor Disruptive Behavior

At the last group meeting, you learned how to reinforce your child's good behavior by using praise. Another effective strategy you can use to manage your child's behavior is to ignore certain behaviors. This entails withdrawing all attention, verbal and physical, from your child's minor disruptive behavior—that is, behavior that is irritating or annoying, but not dangerous. Examples of this type of behavior include whining and begging.

Research shows that talking to a child immediately after he has been caught behaving badly may serve to reward the behavior so the likelihood of it occurring again is higher. Talking, or even reprimanding or scolding, your child can actually increase the likelihood that he will repeat the negative behavior. Some children enjoy getting their parents' attention, regardless of whether it is positive or not. This is why ignoring is an effective technique. When you ignore your child you should cut off all communication with him while the negative behavior is happening. This means not speaking to or looking at your child at all.

Although it sounds easy, ignoring your child is actually very hard to do. This is especially true if your child persists in arguing with you. When you first start to ignore some of your child's minor negative behavior, the frequency of the behavior may actually increase. This is normal and to be expected. It just means that your child is trying harder to get the negative attention he has come to expect. After a while of using the ignoring technique, however, the negative behavior will eventually decrease in frequency. Once you have successfully ended an episode of bad behavior by your child through use of the ignoring technique, it is important for you to look for positive behaviors that you can praise.

Using the Techniques of Praise and Ignoring

Remember the following about using praise:

- Praising your child will increase the likelihood that he will repeat a behavior again.

- Praising your child helps him to develop a positive idea of who he is.

- Praising your child sets a good example for how he should interact with others.

When praising your child you should:

- Maintain good eye contact

- Speak clearly and repeat the praise so that they really do hear you

- Label the behavior that you are praising them for

- Use unlabeled praise when appropriate

- Praise as close in time to the behavior as possible

Remember the following about using ignoring:

- Ignoring bad behavior and paying attention to good behavior go hand-in-hand.

- Paying attention to bad behavior may make the bad behavior worse instead of better.

- Ignoring a bad behavior may make things worse in the beginning, but if you continue to ignore it, the behavior should eventually decrease or go away.

- Ignoring is the opposite of paying attention.

When ignoring your child you should:

- Not look at the child.

- Stop all talking to the child

- Act like you cannot see or hear him

- Leave the room if you need to

- Not give in—keep ignoring the behavior regardless of how long it goes on.

Tracking and Ignoring Your Child's Behavior

Just as you have been tracking your child's behavior and recording your use of praise, you can begin to monitor your use of the ignoring technique. Identify three behaviors that you are willing to practice ignoring and their positive-behavior opposites (see Child Behavior Checklist in chapter 5). Write these behaviors down in the first column of the Praise and Ignoring Behavior Tracking Form at the end of the chapter. Circle whether or not you observed the behaviors and whether you praised or ignored them. Do this for 2 weeks and bring your completed tracking forms to the next group meeting.

Homework

- ✎ Continue monitoring and tracking your child's good behaviors and offer praise when these behaviors occur.

- ✎ Track three negative behaviors and practice ignoring them for 2 weeks with the aid of the Praise and Ignoring Behavior Tracking Form (two copies are provided).

Praise and Ignoring Behavior Tracking Form

BEHAVIOR	Monday	Tuesday	Wednesday	Thursday	Friday	Saturday	Sunday
Neg: _____ _____	Observed Ignored	Observed Ignored	Observed Ignored	Observed Ignored	Observed Ignored	Observed Ignored	Observed Ignored
Pos: _____ _____	Observed Praised	Observed Praised	Observed Praised	Observed Praised	Observed Praised	Observed Praised	Observed Praised
Neg: _____ _____	Observed Ignored	Observed Ignored	Observed Ignored	Observed Ignored	Observed Ignored	Observed Ignored	Observed Ignored
Pos: _____ _____	Observed Praised	Observed Praised	Observed Praised	Observed Praised	Observed Praised	Observed Praised	Observed Praised
Neg: _____ _____	Observed Ignored	Observed Ignored	Observed Ignored	Observed Ignored	Observed Ignored	Observed Ignored	Observed Ignored
Pos: _____ _____	Observed Praised	Observed Praised	Observed Praised	Observed Praised	Observed Praised	Observed Praised	Observed Praised

Praise and Ignoring Behavior Tracking Form

BEHAVIOR	Monday	Tuesday	Wednesday	Thursday	Friday	Saturday	Sunday
Neg: _____ _____	Observed / Ignored	Observed / Ignored	Observed / Ignored	Observed / Ignored	Observed / Ignored	Observed / Ignored	Observed / Ignored
Pos: _____ _____	Observed / Praised	Observed / Praised	Observed / Praised	Observed / Praised	Observed / Praised	Observed / Praised	Observed / Praised
Neg: _____ _____	Observed / Ignored	Observed / Ignored	Observed / Ignored	Observed / Ignored	Observed / Ignored	Observed / Ignored	Observed / Ignored
Pos: _____ _____	Observed / Praised	Observed / Praised	Observed / Praised	Observed / Praised	Observed / Praised	Observed / Praised	Observed / Praised
Neg: _____ _____	Observed / Ignored	Observed / Ignored	Observed / Ignored	Observed / Ignored	Observed / Ignored	Observed / Ignored	Observed / Ignored
Pos: _____ _____	Observed / Praised	Observed / Praised	Observed / Praised	Observed / Praised	Observed / Praised	Observed / Praised	Observed / Praised

Chapter 7

Session 7: Giving Your Child Good Instructions

Goals

- To learn how to give your child good instructions

The Importance of Instructions

Instructions are the *antecedents* to the behaviors of compliance or noncompliance—this is the *A* of the ABC model discussed in Chapter 5; it is what comes before a behavior. It is important for children to learn to follow instructions. Children who cannot or will not comply with their parent's instructions create a negative family climate. This can cause conflict among family members. In addition, if children are not taught to follow directions at home, they may also be noncompliant within multiple settings, including the school, the neighborhood, and the homes of friends. Teachers, parents, and other adults do not enjoy dealing with a child who is noncompliant and defiant. In addition, a child cannot profit from the school environment if she will not follow directions and, as a result, her grades may drop. Other parents will not want the child in their home and, as a result, peer relationships may be affected. Being able to follow adult instructions is a very important skill for children to learn, and it is your responsibility to teach this skill to your child. Some children may not have difficulty following instructions at home but may have difficulty following them at school. If this is the case with your child, you can still work with her on following directions at home as a way of helping your child improve her school behavior.

Instructions that Don't Work

The following are types of ineffective instructions that you should avoid using with your child.

Buried Instructions: Instructions that are followed by too much talking by the parent. The talking usually takes the form of too much explaining and rationalizing about why the task should be done. It can also take the form of a lot of scolding or criticizing after the command is given.

Example: "John, go put on your sweater because it's cold outside. You know how you always get chilled and then you catch a cold. Then you have to stay home from school, and this gets you behind in your schoolwork."

Chain Instructions: Stringing or chaining too many commands together. If more than two commands are given at once, the child may not be able to sustain attention through the entire string. The child may also begin to obey the first command in the string but become distracted and lose track of the later commands in the string.

Example: "Get to you room, and clean up that mess on the floor, and make up your bed, and take out the garbage, and then get in there and fix a sandwich for your little brother."

Questions Instructions: Phrasing the instruction in the form of a question instead of a command. By doing this you convey to the child that he or she has a choice as to whether or not to follow the instruction. Punishing a child for not following an instruction like this (where he or she has been given a choice) is not fair and it elicits further noncompliance.

Example: "Don't you think you should turn off the TV and do your homework now?"

Repeated Instructions: Repeating the same command over and over again. Parents often have a "magic number" that defines how many times they are willing to repeat a command before they reach their limit. After repeated experiences with their parents, children learn the "magic number." This teaches children that they may ignore their parents until the parent begins to get close to her limit. Then and only then does the child have to listen and comply. This kind of experience teaches the child to tune the parent out.

Example: "Take out the garbage. I said, take out the garbage. Didn't you hear me? I said take out the garbage!"

Vague Instructions: Vague commands that are not specific. They do not state exactly what the parent wants the child to do.

Examples:

"Stop that!"

"Behave yourself!"

"Be good."

"Calm down."

"Grow up!"

"Act your age!"

"Let's . . . " Instructions: Commands that begin with "Let's . . . ." These commands imply that the parent and child are going to do the task together when, in fact, the parent wants the child to do the task independently. In addition to conveying a lack of confidence in the child's ability to perform the command independently, these types of instructions elicit noncompliance, probably because the child feels tricked into complying when the parent does not help.

Example: "Let's go clean up your room."

Instructions Yelled from a Distance: This is when the parent yells an instruction to the child from another room in the house. In this scenario, the parent may not be aware of what the child is doing and may be interrupting the child in the middle of a highly absorbing task. In addition, it is more difficult to keep your tone of voice respectful when a command is being yelled from another room. All of these conditions make it less likely that the child will comply with the instruction.

Example: "Emily! I am waiting in the laundry room for you to bring me your clothes! Go to your room and get your clothes right now!" Meanwhile, Emily is heavily engrossed in playing her videogame. She is beating her older brother Al for the very first time, and the two have made a deal: if she wins this game he will take her out for ice cream on Saturday. Unfortunately, Emily hears her mother screaming from down the hall, she becomes upset and loses the game. Emily begins to cry and her brother starts teasing her that she will not get any ice cream on Saturday.

If you are able to give your child good instructions, he or she is more likely to follow them. If you give your child bad or ineffective instructions, he or she is more likely not to follow them. Punishing your child for not following bad instructions is not a good decision. This is why it is so important that you learn to give effective instructions.

Good instructions are

- Direct and specific

- Stated clearly

- Limited to only one or two at a time

- Followed by 10 seconds of silence

An example of a good instruction is as follows:

"Johnny, your room is very messy. Please, go clean it up now."

When giving your child instructions, be sure to keep the following guidelines in mind:

1. Do not give an instruction if you are not willing to follow through with a punishment when your child does not comply.

2. Do not give an instruction that your child does not have the skill or capacity to complete.

3. Respect your child's ongoing activities. Do not give your child an instruction if she is in the middle of something that you have given permission to do. Wait until that activity is completed.

4. Show respect for your child. Use a pleasant (not hostile or sarcastic) tone of voice.

Homework

✎ Begin practicing good instructions this week and watch to see if your child complies. Remember to praise your child for following good instructions.

Chapter 8

Session 8: Establishing Rules and Expectations

Goals

- To establish household rules and expectations for your child

- To begin monitoring your child's adherence to rules and expectations

Behavior Rules and Expectations

This week you will learn about behavior rules and expectations and how to establish them in your household.

It is important to note the difference between rules and expectations. *Behavior rules* refer to behaviors that you would like your child to decrease, whereas *expectations* refer to behaviors that you would like your child to increase and include things like chores.

Examples of behavior rules include the following:

- No hitting

- No cursing

- No name-calling

- No breaking of things

- No rough play in the house

- No arguing

Examples of expectations include the following:

- Making the bed in the morning

- Taking out the garbage

- Feeding the animals

- Cleaning up after dinner

- Cutting the grass

- Completing homework

Following are some important points to remember about rules and expectations:

- Behavior rules and expectations help children learn to do or not do certain behaviors without having to be told every time.

- Behavior rules and expectations are for behaviors that we want children to learn to control themselves, without having to be told every time.

- When behavior rules or expectations are violated there is always an immediate consequence; do not give warnings or second chances!

- It is up to you to decide what consequences you will use to help your child learn to take responsibility for his negative behavior. It is also up to you to decide what rewards will be given for displaying good behavior. Be sure to discuss these rewards and consequences with your child.

Establishing Behavior Rules and Expectations

Behavior Rules

Follow these four steps for setting up behavior rules in your household:

1. Think of two or three (no more than three) behaviors that you would like your child to learn to stop doing or do without having to be told every time. After your child has learned to follow the first two or three rules, you can add more to the list.

2. Put those behaviors in the form of a rule.

3. Write the rules on a piece of paper and place the paper in a prominent place where everyone in the family can see it (e.g., on the refrigerator door).

4. Tell your child that these are the household rules and that they are in effect in the house at all times. Explain to your child that over the course of the next 1 to 2 weeks you will point out times when he is breaking a rule, but that you will not punish him. For example, "Ashley, you just called your brother a name. That is against our behavior rules." This will give your child a chance to learn the rules before the consequences are implemented. After 1 or 2 weeks, your child will get a punishment every time he breaks the rules or does not do what is expected of him.

Expectations

Follow these four steps for setting up household expectations and chores:

1. Think of two or three chores or expectations that you want your child to do every week. Examples include vacuuming or sweeping, taking out the garbage, cleaning his room, helping cook dinner, or doing the dishes.

2. Sit down with your child and ask for his suggestions. You may let your child have some say in what he will do or allow the expectations to change as needed.

3. Tell your child that these are new expectations and chores will be in effect at all times.

4. Explain to your child that over the course of the next 1 to 2 weeks you will point out times when he does not comply with an expectation or complete a chore, but that you will not punish him. For example, "Johnny, you did not put your toys away after you were done playing with them. This is one of your chores and I expect you to do it." This will give your child a chance to get used to your expectations. After this period of pointing out the behaviors, your child will receive a punishment every time he does not do what is expected of him.

✎ Identify three specific behavior rules you would like to institute in your home this week and post them, along with a list of rewards and consequences, some place where all family members can see them. You should include your child in discussion of the development of rules.

✎ Track your child's compliance to the rules over the next 2 weeks using the Behavior Rules Tracking Form at the end of the chapter. Remember, do not use punishment during this period unless your child engages in behavior that is dangerous or harmful.

✎ Establish expectations and track your child's compliance using the Expectations Tracking Form at the end of the chapter. Again, do not punish your child yet for failing to meet expectations or complete chores.

Behavior Rules Tracking Form

BEHAVIOR RULES	Monday	Tuesday	Wednesday	Thursday	Friday	Saturday	Sunday
1. _____ _____	Complied Rewarded Noncompliant Labeled	Complied Rewarded Noncompliant Labeled	Complied Rewarded Noncompliant Labeled	Complied Rewarded Noncompliant Labeled	Complied Rewarded Noncompliant Labeled	Complied Rewarded Noncompliant Labeled	Complied Rewarded Noncompliant Labeled
2. _____ _____	Complied Rewarded Noncompliant Labeled	Complied Rewarded Noncompliant Labeled	Complied Rewarded Noncompliant Labeled	Complied Rewarded Noncompliant Labeled	Complied Rewarded Noncompliant Labeled	Complied Rewarded Noncompliant Labeled	Complied Rewarded Noncompliant Labeled
3. _____ _____	Complied Rewarded Noncompliant Labeled	Complied Rewarded Noncompliant Labeled	Complied Rewarded Noncompliant Labeled	Complied Rewarded Noncompliant Labeled	Complied Rewarded Noncompliant Labeled	Complied Rewarded Noncompliant Labeled	Complied Rewarded Noncompliant Labeled

Behavior Rules Tracking Form

BEHAVIOR RULES	Monday	Tuesday	Wednesday	Thursday	Friday	Saturday	Sunday
1. _No talk back_	Complied	Complied	Complied	Complied	Complied	Complied	Complied
	Rewarded	Rewarded	Rewarded	Rewarded	Rewarded	Rewarded	Rewarded
	Noncompliant	Noncompliant	Noncompliant	Noncompliant	Noncompliant	Noncompliant	Noncompliant
	Labeled	Labeled	Labeled	Labeled	Labeled	Labeled	Labeled
2. _No rude talk_	Complied	Complied	Complied	Complied	Complied	Complied	Complied
	Rewarded	Rewarded	Rewarded	Rewarded	Rewarded	Rewarded	Rewarded
	Noncompliant	Noncompliant	Noncompliant	Noncompliant	Noncompliant	Noncompliant	Noncompliant
	Labeled	Labeled	Labeled	Labeled	Labeled	Labeled	Labeled
3. _No blame others for your rudeness_	Complied	Complied	Complied	Complied	Complied	Complied	Complied
	Rewarded	Rewarded	Rewarded	Rewarded	Rewarded	Rewarded	Rewarded
	Noncompliant	Noncompliant	Noncompliant	Noncompliant	Noncompliant	Noncompliant	Noncompliant
	Labeled	Labeled	Labeled	Labeled	Labeled	Labeled	Labeled

Expectations Tracking Form

EXPECTATIONS	Monday	Tuesday	Wednesday	Thursday	Friday	Saturday	Sunday
1. _____ _____ _____	Complied Rewarded Noncompliant Labeled	Complied Rewarded Noncompliant Labeled	Complied Rewarded Noncompliant Labeled	Complied Rewarded Noncompliant Labeled	Complied Rewarded Noncompliant Labeled	Complied Rewarded Noncompliant Labeled	Complied Rewarded Noncompliant Labeled
2. _____ _____ _____	Complied Rewarded Noncompliant Labeled	Complied Rewarded Noncompliant Labeled	Complied Rewarded Noncompliant Labeled	Complied Rewarded Noncompliant Labeled	Complied Rewarded Noncompliant Labeled	Complied Rewarded Noncompliant Labeled	Complied Rewarded Noncompliant Labeled
3. _____ _____ _____	Complied Rewarded Noncompliant Labeled	Complied Rewarded Noncompliant Labeled	Complied Rewarded Noncompliant Labeled	Complied Rewarded Noncompliant Labeled	Complied Rewarded Noncompliant Labeled	Complied Rewarded Noncompliant Labeled	Complied Rewarded Noncompliant Labeled

Expectations Tracking Form

EXPECTATIONS	Monday	Tuesday	Wednesday	Thursday	Friday	Saturday	Sunday
1. _____	Complied Rewarded Noncompliant Labeled	Complied Rewarded Noncompliant Labeled	Complied Rewarded Noncompliant Labeled	Complied Rewarded Noncompliant Labeled	Complied Rewarded Noncompliant Labeled	Complied Rewarded Noncompliant Labeled	Complied Rewarded Noncompliant Labeled
2. _____	Complied Rewarded Noncompliant Labeled	Complied Rewarded Noncompliant Labeled	Complied Rewarded Noncompliant Labeled	Complied Rewarded Noncompliant Labeled	Complied Rewarded Noncompliant Labeled	Complied Rewarded Noncompliant Labeled	Complied Rewarded Noncompliant Labeled
3. _____	Complied Rewarded Noncompliant Labeled	Complied Rewarded Noncompliant Labeled	Complied Rewarded Noncompliant Labeled	Complied Rewarded Noncompliant Labeled	Complied Rewarded Noncompliant Labeled	Complied Rewarded Noncompliant Labeled	Complied Rewarded Noncompliant Labeled

Chapter 9

Session 9: Discipline and Punishment—Part I

Goals

- To learn about punishment and how to use it properly and effectively

- To review the concepts of the time-out technique

Discipline and Punishment

So far in this program, you have learned how to use praise and ignoring to manage your child's behavior. You have also learned how to give your child good instructions and how to establish behavior rules and expectations. This week, you will learn about punishment.

The focus of group for the next 2 weeks is establishing behavior rules and expectations for your child. Although the group will discuss punishment this week, you should not implement any of the punishment strategies discussed until your child has had sufficient time to adjust to the new rules and expectations you have established.

We hope that you have seen some improvement in your child's behavior by this point. However, most children will not improve enough by using only positive strategies and, as a result, other strategies are needed. For behaviors that are nonresponsive to positive strategies or cannot be dealt with effectively through use of the ignoring technique, parents need to use punishment procedures.

Punishment is the occurrence of a negative or unpleasant event following a particular negative behavior. Effective punishment decreases the frequency of the behavior in the future. In contrast, *positive reinforcement*, in which a positive (pleasant) event follows a behavior, results in an increase in the frequency of that behavior in the future.

Following are some examples of effective punishment (and non-punishment) in everyday life:

- Jeremy fights with his little brother and is grounded for the weekend—no TV, no phone calls, and no games. Jeremy does not fight with his little brother again or the frequency of fighting decreases.

- Paul is late for football practice and the coach keeps him out of the game for the first quarter. Paul is never late for football practice again.

Following are some examples of ineffective punishment:

- Jason hits his little brother. His mother yells at him and tells him never to do this again. Jason hits his brother again the next day and every day after that for the next week. His mother yells at him every time he hits his brother. Jason stops hitting his brother at the moment his mother yells at him, but he does it again every day.

The "punishment" in this last example is ineffective because the behavior (hitting his brother) actually increases. Therefore, it is not really punishment, even though the mother may intend it to be punishment. To be an effective punishment, the negative consequence should result in a decrease or total elimination of the bad behavior.

Sometimes parents think that something they do is punishment because it stops the child's behavior at that moment. This includes yelling, screaming, or otherwise verbally reprimanding your child. If your child continues to do the behavior day after day, then what you are doing is not really punishment—it is not working to teach your child to stop doing the behavior in the long run.

Punishment Concepts

Severe Punishment

Following are reasons why you should minimize the use of severe punishment, verbal or physical.

1. **People avoid others who punish them**. No one likes to be hit or criticized. So we try to stay away from people who might hit or criticize us. If you severely punish your child, and do this often, she will probably try to stay away from you.

2. **The methods you use to punish your child teach her how to punish others.** Children who are severely punished tend to be more aggressive with other children; this is especially true when the child is punished on a frequent basis. In addition, these children may grow up to be aggressive adults.

3. **Excessive use of punishment lowers your child's self-esteem and results in them losing any motivation to change behavior.** You should always try to control your child's behavior with rewards first. There are some times, however, when the use of punishment is necessary, although physical punishment is not recommended.

Moderate Punishment

You may have to use moderate punishment in the following cases.

1. **When the problem behavior may cause the child to hurt herself or others.** For example, you do not want to stand around and watch your child play with fire until she learns a lesson. Instead, you may have to use punishment to stop this behavior before your child gets burned.

2. **When your rewards do not work because other stronger rewards encourage the problem behavior.** You cannot control the rewards your child receives outside of the home (e.g., playing with other children), so you make a rule such as the following: "For every minute after such and such time that you are late, you go to bed 5 minutes earlier."

3. **When noncompliance continues at high rates even after rewards have been instituted for compliance.**

1. **Punish immediately.** If you wait an hour to punish your child for hitting her brother she may think she is getting punished for something else done in the meantime. She may never make the connection between hitting her brother and being punished.

2. **Be calm, rational, and matter-of-fact.** If you get angry and yell or scream or criticize your child while you are punishing her, you are likely to cause your child to resent you and hate you for the moment.

3. **Do not "give in."** Rewards should never be given for behaviors you want to stop. For example, you want your children to stop throwing tantrums when they do not get their way. Usually you ignore them for doing this. But sometimes you give in and give them what they want. This practice rewards them for throwing tantrums. So they will continue to have tantrums, hoping that sometimes they will get you to give in. If you really want them to stop the tantrums, punish them every time this happens. This behavior will stop much faster than if you punish them some times and reward them other times.

4. **Give a warning signal.** If you must use punishment to control your child's behavior, it is best to give them a warning signal first. Soon the warning will be enough to make your child stop misbehaving.

5. **Make it brief.** Long lectures often reduce the effectiveness of punishment; the same is true for extended periods of grounding. Long lectures may make parents feel better, but they do not usually decrease children's misbehavior. Parents may threaten long periods of grounding when they are angry, but then they often do not follow through with the long grounding. Keep your statements specific and short.

Good punishment is used along with rewards for other positive behaviors. If you reward your children a great deal for positive behavior, they will learn that they do not have to misbehave to get your attention. They can get your attention when they behave.

You are probably familiar with time-out, and you may even have experience using it with your own child. A *time-out* means taking time out from positive reinforcement. The procedure requires quickly removing your child from anything that is positive (e.g., TV, a nice view, books, other people, etc.) whenever a particular misbehavior occurs. When you remove your child from positive stimuli, you must be silent, because talking is considered something positive to the child and will actually act to reinforce or increase the likelihood that your child will engage again in the same behavior for which she is being placed in time-out.

For fourth, fifth, and sixth graders, the best place to conduct a time-out is in the bathroom, laundry room, or any other room of the house devoid of entertainment. Time-out should never take place in the child's room or in any other room where there are interesting or fun things to do (e.g., watch TV, play games, etc.).

Time-out should be used for *noncompliance to good instructions* and for *violations of behavior rules*.

Steps for Time-out for Noncompliance

1. Give a good instruction.

2. Wait for 10 seconds. Do not talk during the 10 seconds.

3. If your child does not follow instructions within the 10 seconds, give a warning: "If you do not do ＿＿＿＿＿＿＿ , you will have to go to time-out."

4. Wait for 10 seconds *again*. Do not talk during the 10 seconds.

5. If your child still does not follow instructions within the 10 seconds, say, "Since you did not do ＿＿＿＿＿＿＿ , you have to go to time-out now."

6. Your child should go to your identified time-out place and stay there for 10–20 minutes.

7. *Ignore* your child while she is in time-out. Do not talk to your child, no matter what she says.

8. At the end of the time-out, take your child back to the original situation and give the same instruction again. If she still does not follow instructions, go through the preceding steps *again*. Keep cycling through the steps until the child eventually does what you asked her to do. Keep doing this no matter how long it takes. Your child will learn that you do not intend to back down.

Steps for Time-out for Behavior Rules Violations

If your child violates one of your behavior rules, she gets no warning. There is an immediate time-out. The steps are as follows:

1. Say, "Since you did _____ , and that is against our behavior rules, you have to go to time-out now."

2. The child must go to the time-out place and stay there for 10–20 minutes.

3. *Ignore* your child completely while she is in the time-out place.

4. After time-out is over, take your child back to the original situation and instruct her to repair what she did, apologize to the other person involved, or do some good behavior that is the opposite of the rule that she broke.

Additional Considerations

If your child does not want to go to time-out or tries to come out of the time-out place before time is up, you may try the following:

- Remove a privilege

- Start the timer over again

- Increase the length of the time-out

It is important to remember that if you choose to remove a privilege, that privilege should be something important to the child.

Remember that after taking a time-put, the child is then brought back to the original situation and given the same instruction again to which she must comply, or she will keep going back to time-out. In this way, the child does not "get away with" the misbehavior.

If your child is destructive on the way to the time-out place (e.g., overturns a table), ignore it at the moment and proceed with the time-out for the original misbehavior. Then, take your child back to the area of destruction and tell her to fix it or put it back the way it was. Your child does not get out of punishment for the original misbehavior, and does not get away with the destructive behavior.

If necessary, you may remove all positive or interesting items from the environment where your child is, rather than remove your child from the environment to a time-out place. This is an acceptable alternative only if you can truly remove *all* the positive reinforcers.

Homework

✎ Finalize your time-out procedure and complete the Time-out Worksheet at the end of the chapter and bring it to the next group meeting.

Dec. 13
To practice until next Wednesday

Time-out Worksheet

1. List of behaviors that will result in time-out:

_____

_____

_____

_____

2. Number of warnings before time-out is given: _____

3. Location of time-out: _____

4. Length of time-out: _____

    a. Initial length: _____

    b. Maximum length: _____

5. Rules in time-out:

_____

_____

_____

_____

6. Type of timer to be used: _____

7. Consequences for failure to take a time-out, or failure to follow rules in time-out:

_____

_____

_____

Remember that your child is "off limits" to all family members during time-out. Do not engage in conversation with your child about whether or not they should have a time-out, how long it should be, whether they enjoy time-outs, whether time-out is just a game, and the like.

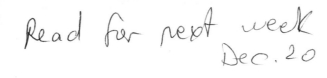

Chapter 10

Session 10: Discipline and Punishment—Part II

Goals

■ To learn different punishment techniques

Privilege Removal

Another approach to effective punishment is something called "privilege removal." This involves quickly taking away a privilege when your child breaks a rule or doesn't follow instructions. For example, if your child does not complete his homework, he cannot have the privilege of watching TV. If your child does not remove his dirty dishes from the table, he cannot have any dessert or evening snacks. If your child hits another child, he is not allowed to go outside and play with friends for one day. The privileges that are removed should be things that your child likes or values, and, if possible, the privilege should be logically related to the misbehavior.

It is important to note that privilege removal should be administered as soon as possible after the misbehavior and should be time limited. The time limit should be clearly articulated to the child at the time that the punishment is imposed (e.g., no TV until the homework is done, no snacks for one night).

Privilege removal can be used for noncompliance with good instructions and violations of behavior rules, just like the time-out procedure discussed in Session 9.

Steps for Privilege Removal for Noncompliance

1. Give a good instruction.

2. Wait for 10 seconds. Do not talk during the 10 seconds.

3. If your child does not follow instructions in the 10 seconds, give a warning: "If you do not do _____, you will lose _____ (privilege)."

4. Wait 10 seconds again. Do not talk during the 10 seconds.

5. If your child still does not follow instructions within the 10 seconds, say, "Since you did not do _____, so you have lost _____ (privilege)."

6. Immediately remove the privilege that has been lost.

7. Give the same instruction and complete the entire sequence using a second privilege.

8. If the child still refuses, the removal of individual privileges should be changed to a total reward shutdown. That is, the child loses *all* privileges if he remains noncompliant with the request (see section on total reward shutdown later in the chapter for more information).

9. *Immediately* put total reward shutdown into effect. Remove access to TV, computer, videogames, iPod, friends, etc.

10. Ignore your child's protests and do not get pulled into an argument with him.

11. Your child comes off of total reward shutdown as soon as he completes the instructions you gave. Thus, it is up to the child how long he remains on total reward shutdown. All the child has to do to get off it is to complete the original instruction. However, if he stubbornly refuses to complete the instruction for several minutes or hours, that is how long the child remains on total reward shutdown.

12. Even if the child eventually completes the instruction and comes off total reward shutdown, the child still loses the first and second privileges because he did not follow your instructions at first.

The goal of this procedure is to teach your child that it is in his best interest to follow your instructions the first time you give them.

Steps for Privilege Removal for Behavior Rules Violations

If your child violates one of your behavior rules, he gets no warning. There is an immediate privilege removal. Your child has already been given 2 weeks to learn these rules and has been told that violations will be met with immediate consequences. You must follow through with your punishment strategy immediately and you must be consistent.

Work Chores

As an alternative to the removal of privileges, assignment of a work chore can also be used as an effective approach to punishment. This means that the child has to do an unpleasant chore as a consequence of his negative behavior. Examples of work chores are numerous but include things like cutting the grass, picking weeds, cleaning a bathroom, and the like. It is important that the work chore not be a job that your child is expected to do anyway. If one of the household expectations is that your child keeps his bathroom clean, you shouldn't make cleaning the bathroom a punishment for negative behavior. Work chores used for punishment purposes are extra work chores that your child would not ordinarily have to do.

Steps for Work Chores for Noncompliance

1. Give a clear instruction.

2. Wait for 10 seconds. Do not talk during the 10 seconds.

3. If your child does not follow instructions in the 10 seconds, give a warning: "If you do not do _____, you will have to _____ (work chore)."

4. Wait for 10 more seconds. Do not talk to the child during the 10 seconds.

5. If your child still does not follow instructions within the 10 seconds, say, "Since you did not do _____, you now have to _____ (work chore)."

6.   After the child does the work chore, give the original instruc-
     tion all over again. Repeat the sequence again, until the child
     follows the original instruction.

Additional Considerations

1.   If your child refuses to do the work chore, issue a warning that
     if he does not follow the original instruction and complete the
     two work chores right away, he will go on total reward shut-
     down (see section on total reward shutdown later in the chap-
     ter for more information). Wait 10 seconds.

2.   If your child does not do what you said within the 10 seconds,
     implement a total reward shutdown. That means taking away
     all of the child's privileges. Do this *immediately*. Do not wait.
     Tell your child that he can come off total reward shutdown as
     soon as he does the original task and the work chore that was
     assigned. **DO NOT ARGUE WITH YOUR CHILD.**

3.   Be sure to follow through with giving back privileges as soon as
     the child completes the two tasks.

Total Reward Shutdown

As mentioned, a total reward shutdown means taking away all of the
child's privileges. This means the child cannot listen to the radio or
iPod, cannot play videogames, watch TV, go out and play or hang
out with other children, or go on any special outings; in general, the
child cannot have any of the privileges that he is used to having. The
child can easily get all of these privileges back by doing the work
chores that he refused to do, as well as the original task that the parent asked the child to do. In this way, total reward shutdown is
different from the usual way that grounding is done. By submitting
to the parents' control and doing the things that the child was asked
to do, the child can get off total reward shutdown. Unlike grounding, this procedure places the child in control of when he will get the
privileges back.

If a child engages in really dangerous or disrespectful behavior such as cursing at the parent, stealing, or threatening others, it may be necessary to give a stronger punishment than the ones just discussed. Serious misbehaviors should be handled with more severe forms of punishment. This does not mean, however, that a person must use physical punishment. Instead, you may choose to assign longer or more difficult work chores (e.g., cleaning the whole garage, raking the entire yard and bagging all the leaves, scrubbing down all the walls in several rooms in the house) or issue a grounding for a pre-scribed, but not too lengthy, period of time. The use of lengthy or unspecified periods of grounding is not recommended because the child may feel that he is in such a deep hole that there is no motiva-tion to change the behavior.

Homework

✎ Complete the Privilege Removal Worksheet at the end of the chapter and post it some place where all family members can view it.

✎ Also complete the Work Chores Worksheet at the end of the chapter and post it for all family members to see.

Privilege Removal Worksheet

Complete this form and post it where all family members can see it. You may photocopy it from the book instead of ripping it out.

Child's Name: _____ Date: _____

Behaviors that Result in Privilege Removal	Privileges to Be Removed
1. Yelling and talking back	- no phone at school for that day - don't give her any attention
2. Blaming others and not taking responsabilities for their behaviours	- no phone - no TV.
3. No finish homework in time	- no TV - earlier bed time
4.	
5.	

Work Chores Worksheet

Complete this form and post it where all family members can see it. You may photocopy it from the book instead of ripping it out.

Child's Name: _____ Date: _____

Behaviors that Result in Work Chores
1.
2.
3.
4.
5.

Possible Chores that May Be Given Are:

_____   _____

_____   _____

_____   _____

_____   _____

_____   _____

Chapter 11

Session 11: Getting Ready for Summer

Goals

- To plan activities to keep your child occupied during the summer

- To celebrate the successful completion of Year 1 of the Coping Power Program

Planning for Summer

Session 11 is the last group meeting before the summer break. Your child has completed school for the year and is no doubt looking forward to the upcoming vacation. Many children like to have unstructured time, to sleep late, and basically do "whatever comes up" during the summer months. However, by the middle of the summer, it is often the case that children are bored and need more productive things to do to keep them busy, occupied, and out of trouble. The more occupied children are with constructive activities, the more likely they are to not get into trouble, not cause problems with brothers and sisters, and so forth. In addition, most teachers and schools encourage children to not completely forget about learning over the summer, but to be involved in some kind of academically oriented activity. Children who stay involved in activities related to learning of academic or vocational skills (e.g., reading, writing, drama, music) over the summer tend to do better in class when school resumes in the fall.

Daily Structure

After the first couple of weeks of no schedule and watching TV, most children profit from some kind of daily structure in their summer schedules. Parents will vary with regard to how much structure they wish to introduce. For some parents and children, a daily calendar that lists activities for the day in the relevant time slots as well as any chores or expectations that the parent has for the child is useful. Such activities and chores may be written in on an hour-by-hour basis. For other parents enough structure is provided by writing the day's activities on a blackboard, as well as what chores the child must complete before the outing or activity can be done. However, regardless of the method you choose, some sort of communication with your child on a daily basis is a good idea for virtually all children this age.

Activities for Parents and Children Together

For parents who are able to be home with their children during the day or for at least part of the day, doing something together can be one way to enjoy the summer and break up a long day. Your group leader may provide you with a resource guide of fun things to do in your community.

Community-Based Activities and Events

Family outings outside of home are another option for introducing structure into the long summer weeks and months. There are many community events that are available to children and families at no cost or relatively low cost. You may refer to the resource guide (if you received one) or check your local newspapers for upcoming events.

Reading Program for the Summer

Most teachers recommend that children continue to read on a daily basis throughout the summer. This is especially important for elementary and early middle school students, who are still consolidating their reading skills. The public libraries are very user-friendly, and librarians are happy to assist parents in finding age- and grade-appropriate reading materials for their children. Some libraries even have charts and ideas for reward programs to help motivate children to read over the summer. Many libraries also have summer read-aloud programs in which librarians read aloud to groups of children.

Summer Chores

If children have some daily chores to do over the summer they have an opportunity to practice the kind of daily responsibility that is so important in school, where they have daily expectations for performing tasks and homework, etc. Children who have some daily chores built into their summer schedules generally make a better transition back into the responsibilities of school and homework in the fall.

Children at Home Alone During the Day

Many children have to spend some time at home alone or in the charge of older siblings during the day in the summer months. For these children it is even more important that daily structure be put into place in a pre-planned way, since parents are not available in person to provide structure on a minute-to-minute basis.

Surviving Family Vacations

Provide as much structure as possible when on a family vacation so that your child knows what to expect and what is expected of her. Giving your child an itinerary with estimations of how long it will take to get to the vacation destination is helpful. This way, your child can set her own expectations.

For long car rides, taking along play materials that children can occupy themselves with in the car is a must. Books on tape or on CD are another great idea. Most libraries now have children's books on tape or CD that can be played in the car cassette or CD player or in the child's portable tape or CD player. One children's writer has recommended that, on long car rides, each child have their own portable tape or CD player to listen to their own audiobook. This way each child is occupied with a developmentally appropriate and interesting activity, and the parents are free to have an adult conversation or listen to their own music or book on tape.

Playing family games in the car can be a way to draw the family together in a fun way during a long car ride. For example, you can play the "state game," where you "collect states" by spotting them on license plates. You can also reduce boredom by stopping for short breaks so everyone can stretch their legs or do some fun side activities along the way.

Staying with Noncustodial Parents over the Summer

Some children may be spending significant amounts of time with the non-custodial parent over the summer. If this applies to your family, there are several issues you may want to consider. For example, it is important to try to maintain the structure that has been put in place for your child in your home across both households. Your child will also benefit from consistency across both households with regard to rules, chores, expectations, etc. For this to be possible, both parents (and any step-parents) need to communicate openly with one another.

Dealing with Increased Levels of Stress

There is a possibility that you will experience higher stress levels during the summer months as your work and personal lives continue while the structure and routines of the school year come to an abrupt end. In addition to the stresses you normally experience, you will have the added stress of providing structure, supervision, and monitoring for your child during the daytime hours, as well as dealing with increases of troublesome behavior that can occur for children when structure decreases.

Despite the perception that summer is a time for "fun and relaxation," being a parent can actually be more difficult and stressful during the summer. In order to deal with summer stress, "taking care of yourself" as an individual is one of the most important things you can do. Taking some individual time for yourself and getting away from work, parenting, and household problems (even if it is just for 30 minutes a day), is a good place to start. If you can take a few days of "adult vacation" by yourself or with a spouse, companion, or friend (without children), this may be a good idea as well. All adults can benefit from getting away from the daily demands placed on them in the various roles in their lives. Refer back to your Pie Chart of Life (see Chapter 3). Look at how much time you are dedicating to other areas of your life, instead of devoting time to taking care of yourself. Making time for yourself can actually reduce your overall stress level giving you more energy to deal with your other roles when you come back.

Homework

✎ Review Chapters 3 and 4 and the different ways you can manage your stress. Use these strategies over the summer break.

✎ Take care of yourself!

Coping Power Parent Program
Year 2

Chapter 12

Session 12: Academic Support in the Home: Review Session—Year 2

Goals

- To get reacquainted with the group and start Year 2 of the Coping Power Program

- To review last year's topic, providing your child with academic support at home

- To reestablish a homework system

Welcome Back

Welcome back to the Coping Power Program! Congratulate yourself on returning to the group and wanting to continue to improve your parenting skills and help your child cope with the start of a new school year.

Your first group meeting of the year will serve as a review of last year's topic, providing academic support in the home.

Review of Academic Support in the Home

As discussed last year, there are many things you can do in the home to support your child's academic success, especially completion of homework assignments. Remember the homework system you established last year? It is important to review this system, now that your child is starting a new school year and entering middle school. The emphasis on homework increases significantly as students move from elementary to secondary school. Establishing good homework and study habits early in the year can help to prevent students from getting so far behind in their homework that they become discouraged or give up entirely.

If last year's homework system worked for you and your child, you should reinstate it this year. Remember to get input from your child's teacher to develop a system that works for all those involved (you, your child, and the teacher). Like last year, you may want to set up a parent–teacher conference to enlist the teacher's help in establishing a method for monitoring homework. You may wish to ask the teacher if he is willing to initial your child's list of homework assignments before the end of each school day to indicate that all items are listed correctly. Refer to the list of questions for a parent–teacher conference in Chapter 2.

Homework System Forms

Again, we have provided examples of forms at the end of the chapter that you may wish to use when establishing your homework system. You may have used these forms last year. Please feel free to photocopy them from the book or use them as models for creating your own.

Some schools have moved to a Web-based system in which teachers post daily homework assignments and parents can check the postings to find out exactly what the homework is for each class. If your school has such as system, we encourage you to check on your child's homework postings each night as a way of accurately monitoring his assignments.

Spouses and Significant Others

The topic of the next parent group meeting is building family cohesion and improving family functioning. You are encouraged to bring your spouse or significant other to the session, as he or she will benefit from the discussion as well.

Homework

✎ Reinstate a homework system. Review chapters 1 and 2 of the workbook if you need help remembering what to do.

✎ Invite a guest to next week's meeting.

My Homework Plan

I, _____ , agree to the homework plan outlined below.

I will:

- Decide when and where I will do my homework. For example, I will pick a quiet place in the house and pick a time of day to always do my homework.

- Make sure I have all the things I need before starting my homework. For example, I will make sure that I have pencils, paper, erasers, or anything else I may need.

- Always put away everything else that I do not need

- Not do my homework in front of the television or while listening to the radio

- Not talk on the phone during the time I have put aside to complete my homework

- Work on big projects by breaking them down into smaller, more manageable pieces. I will work on the smaller pieces each day.

- Always double-check my answers

- Always ask mom or dad to check my homework and make sure that I have completed everything

- Place notes to remind myself of what I need to do. I will put these notes in a place where I will see them (e.g., my locker, notebook, or desk).

I will do my homework at _____ (time) and I will do it in the _____ (place). If I need to change this schedule, I will talk to mom or dad first.

I will ask _____ to check my homework when I am finished.

Signed: _____ Date: _____

Homework Tracking Form—Teacher Version

Dear parent,

Your child, _____ , is missing the following assignments in:

Math (Teacher signature : _____)

_____

_____

Social Studies (Teacher signature : _____)

_____

_____

Language (Teacher signature : _____)

_____

_____

Science (Teacher signature : _____)

_____

_____

Health (Teacher signature : _____)

_____

_____

Reading (Teacher signature : _____)

_____

_____

Other _____ (Teacher signature : _____)

_____

_____

_____

Chapter 13

Session 13: Building Family Cohesion

Goals

- To learn to improve family functioning by participating in activities that are fun and enjoyable for everyone

Improving Family Functioning

There are many things you can do to improve the cohesiveness and overall functioning of your family. Provided here is just a small sampling of practices that are found to work.

- Get involved with your kids! Go to sporting events and all extracurricular activities with them.

- Talk to your kids in a nonjudgmental and open manner.

- Nurture your relationship with your children. Don't forget to spend time alone with them on a regular basis.

- Establish clear expectations and rules.

- Make consequences for misbehavior known to everyone and follow through with them on a consistent basis.

- Keep conflict to a minimum by creating a positive environment. This means "catching your children being good," or noticing and praising their good behavior at least as often as you catch them being disruptive.

- Teach your kids to problem solve with words and not violence.

- Negotiate with your children when you can.

- Do not abuse alcohol or substances. Your emotional availability and ability to monitor, reward, and discipline your child decrease substantially if you are abusing alcohol or mood-altering substances. If you can't stop by yourself, consider seeking treatment.

▪ Talk to your child about their future and help them to plan.

Building Family Cohesion

Building family cohesion means to build a warm and supportive atmosphere where you and your family can have positive experiences with one another, both inside and outside of the home.

Family Cohesion Inside the Home

Think of some activities that your family can engage in at home that will create fun or pleasant experiences for everyone. It is important that these activities be fun for everyone, especially your child. Be sure to include your child when choosing activities for your family. Ask your child for ideas of fun things your family can do together.

One example of a planned family event is a "family night," when families stay at home and engage in an activity together, such as playing card or board games, reading stories or a novel, baking cookies, watching a scary movie, etc.

Alternatively, instead of establishing a family night, some families try to spend small amounts of time together over the course of the week and on weekends. For example, some families sit down together at the kitchen table for 30 minutes, four times a week, and talk or play a game together. Figure out what works best for you and your family.

Family Cohesion Outside of the Home

In addition to positive family experiences at home, it is also possible to have positive family experiences outside of the home. Some of these, such as going to the circus or a movie or playing miniature golf, require financial resources, while others are relatively inexpensive activities that families can take part in, such as going to the mall, taking a walk or riding bikes around the neighborhood, or having a picnic at a local park. It is not the cost of the activity that matters, only that you and your family enjoy yourselves and have fun together.

Use the worksheet at the end of the chapter to list ideas of fun activities that your family will enjoy.

Homework

 ✎ If not done during the session, complete the Family Cohesion Worksheet and commit to engaging in family activities both inside and outside of the home.

Family Cohesion Worksheet

"In-Home" Activities That We Can Do as a Family: **How Often We Can Do This:**

_____   _____

_____   _____

_____   _____

_____   _____

_____   _____

_____   _____

"Out-of-Home" Activities That We Can Do as a Family: **How Often We Can Do This:**

_____   _____

_____   _____

_____   _____

_____   _____

_____   _____

_____   _____

Chapter 14

Session 14: Family Problem Solving

Family Problem Solving

There may be times when two or more people in your family have a conflict or a difference of opinion about something and they need to find a way to resolve the conflict so that the problem doesn't get worse. Think about your family and some of the problems you may be seeing at home, between either you and your child, your child and his siblings, or you and your spouse or significant other.

When a problem or conflict arises, it is often helpful to use problem solving to resolve the issue.

Steps of Family Problem Solving

If your child is participating in the Coping Power Program, he or she is currently learning about problem solving, so it is important that you to understand the process as well. The problem-solving model is called the "PICC model" and involves the following four steps:

Step 1. Problem Identification

Perspective Taking

- Identify what the problem is, based on **each** persons' perspective of the situation.

- Be as objective as possible in labeling what the problem is and don't use blaming, name-calling, or put-downs in stating the problem.

Individual Goals

- Identify your goal in the situation.

- Identity the other person's goal in the situation.

- Look toward cooperation and compromise.

Step 2. Identify Choices

- Brainstorm all possible solutions.

- Do not evaluate the solutions in terms of outcome but simply list all possible choices.

Step 3. Identify Consequences

- Identify what the consequences would be for each solution.

- Provide *all* possible consequences, both positive and negative.

Step 4. Choose the Best Solution

- Choose the best solution based on a review of all the consequences.

- Weigh the positives and negatives and go with the solution that has the fewest negatives.

- Implement that solution.

- Choose a backup solution in case the first solution does not work and implement the second solution if necessary.

Your group leader will discuss the PICC model in more detail at this week's meeting.

Homework

✎ Hold a family meeting to discuss the problem-solving (PICC) model.

✎ Commit to using the model to try resolving one ongoing conflict at home.

✎ Use the Problem-Solving Worksheet to monitor your use of the problem-solving method when resolving conflicts with your child.

Problem-Solving Worksheet

We agree on the following definition of the problem:

_____

_____

_____

Possible choices: Consequences of the choices:

_____   _____

_____   _____

_____   _____

_____   _____

_____   _____

_____   _____

The solution we have chosen is:

_____

_____

_____

We will implement this solution for week(s) and then talk about how it is working.

Signature of Child:

_____

Signature of Parent:

_____

Chapter 15

Session 15: Family Communication

Family Communication over the Long Term

The skills that you are learning now will be helpful in developing and maintaining a harmonious family environment and will help you to meet the challenges associated with parenting during your child's adolescent years.

As your child gets older and enters adolescence, the way you will accomplish certain goals will change because your child has new developmental needs. For example, right now, you may have a rule that your child has to be in the house by dark on weekends. However, in the future, as she gets older, your child may want to renegotiate her curfew. As the parent, you will probably still want to have a rule about curfew, but you will need to negotiate the actual details.

Parenting is an evolving process that changes and adapts to meet the needs of developing children. Think about how your role as a parent will change as your child gets older and how you will respond to the needs of your developing child.

Structuring Family Communication

Family meetings are one way to respond to the changing needs of your child. Family meetings can serve to continue positive parent involvement in children's lives and to prevent problems in the future.

Family meetings can be used to:

- Develop plans for spending positive family time together

- Discuss problems that have arisen in the family

- Review the rules, expectations, and consequences for behavior

- Negotiate with children about their requests for special privileges

- Revise the household rules

Following are some ideas for setting up family meetings:

- Schedule family meetings on a regular basis.

- Make mealtime a time for the whole family to sit down together and talk.

- Have everyone write down their concerns and bring them to the family meeting.

- Hang a bulletin board or chalkboard in a central location for family members to write down agenda items.

- Give children permission to come to the parent on an "as-needed" basis to discuss concerns.

- Circulate an "invitation" to each family member. The invitation should have basic information such as date, time, and place of the next meeting and include spaces on which people can write their agenda items. Each person should bring the invitation to the meeting. You may use the template provided to create your invitations.

As children get older, one of the ways they will begin to assert their independence is by requesting to go out with their friends (without adult supervision). During these times, family communication is even more important. As the parent, you need to be able to monitor your child's activity, even though you won't be present. By telling you who she is going out with, what they are going to do, where they will be, when they will leave and when they will be home, and how they will get to and from the activity, your child is forced to actually make these plans and to communicate them to you. In this way, you can monitor the people and activities that your child is engaged with.

The form on page 104 can be helpful in making sure that your child keeps you informed of her schedule. You may photocopy the form from the book or use it as a model for creating your own.

You're Invited!

What: Family Meeting

Where: _____

               _____

When: _____

               _____

Our Agenda: _____

               _____

               _____

               _____

               _____

Four W's and an H!

To be completed by the child and presented to the parent *before* all outings.

1. WHO I will be with:

_____

_____

_____

2. WHAT I will be doing:

_____

_____

_____

3. WHERE I will be (including phone number):

_____

_____

_____

4. WHEN I will come home:

_____

_____

_____

5. HOW I will get to and from my destination:

_____

_____

_____

Signature: _____ Date: _____

Homework

✏ Talk with your family about ways of improving and maintaining open communication with one another.

✏ Try to set up at least one family meeting before the next group session.

Chapter 16

Session 16: The End of the Coping Power Program

Planning for the Long Term

Now that the Coping Power Program is ending, it is important to think about planning for the long term. There are many resources available to you and your child, both in the school and in the community.

School Resources for Your Child

Work with your group leader to complete the resource chart provided on page 108. Use it to list the various programs that may be offered at your child's school. Because programs frequently change, you may wish to contact the school principal or guidance counselor for more information.

Community Resources for the Child and Family

Most cities have a selection of private and government-sponsored services to assist families with a variety of problems and concerns. Ask your group leader for a list of these resources, if available.

Program Review

For your reference, we have provided a copy of the Coping Power Program curriculum on page 109. Review the curriculum and talk to your group leader if you have any questions or concerns about any of the topics listed.

School	Peer Mediation Program	After-School Programs	Tutors	Sports Programs	School Counselors	School Social Workers

Table 16.1 Coping Power Program-Parent Group Curriculum

Session	Description
Year 1	
1	Introductions, Overview, and Academic Support
2	Academic Support in the Home
3–4	Stress Management
5	Basic Social Learning Theory and Improving the Parent-Child Relationship
6	Ignoring Minor Disruptive Behavior
7	Giving Effective Instructions to Children
8	Establishing Rules and Expectations
9–10	Discipline and Punishment
11	Getting Ready for Summer
Year 2	
12	Academic Support in the Home-Review Session
13	Family Cohesion Building
14	Family Problem Solving
15	Family Communication
16	The End of the Coping Power Program

The End

Congratulations! You have successfully completed the Coping Power parent training program. We hope that you have benefited from your involvement in this program and that your child has shown positive improvements in his behavior and academic performance.

Being a parent is a lifelong task and the skills you have learned throughout this program will help both you and your child for years to come. It will probably be important to continue to use the skills learned in this program for some time to come in order to help your child continue the improvements he has made in the program. It is especially important to reinstitute procedures at the beginning of each school year (e.g., meeting with the new teacher, establishing a method for tracking homework assignments, setting up homework structures and rules) so that your child gets off to a good start at the beginning of each new academic year. Likewise, continuing to reward and praise your child for good behavior and have consistent discipline for negative behavior remain important throughout childhood and adolescence.

Remember to adapt and modify these skills as necessary in order to respond to your child's changing needs. For example, as your child gets older, the way you carry out punishment may change (e.g., time-out is not appropriate to use with a 15-year-old, but response cost and contingent work chores are appropriate punishments for teens). Likewise, you may not use trips to the park as a reward with an older teen but substitute use of the family car for a specified activity instead. Just remember that the ABC principles of behavior are the same even though some of the specific strategies may change. You can use these principles and adapted strategies up until your child is ready to leave home, taking his developmental level into account as he gets older. Continued use of parenting knowledge acquired in this program will reap rewards in the form of better behavior from your child and pride in yourself for working hard at being a good parent.

Printed in the USA/Agawam, MA
May 26, 2016

635348.005